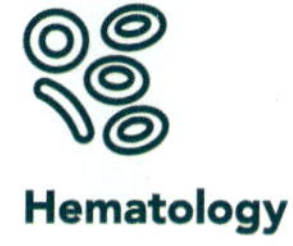

Hematology

First, the facts...

1 Alpha thalassemia (AT) is a blood condition you are born with. You have to inherit a gene change from both parents to have AT.

2 If you inherit a gene change from one parent, you are a carrier but don't have the condition. If your partner is also a carrier, you have a chance of having a child with AT.

3 AT is most common in people with ancestry from Southeast and South Asia, Africa, the Middle East and around the Mediterranean.

4 There are two pairs of genes involved in AT – you may have one, two, three or four gene changes. There are also different types of gene changes – the gene can either be missing or damaged.

5 How severe your AT is depends on the number and type of gene changes you have.

6 AT major (four gene changes) is typically fatal before or shortly after birth without intervention. It remains a lifelong condition but can now be managed with treatment.

This booklet helps you understand AT so that you can talk to your medical team about your condition and its treatment.

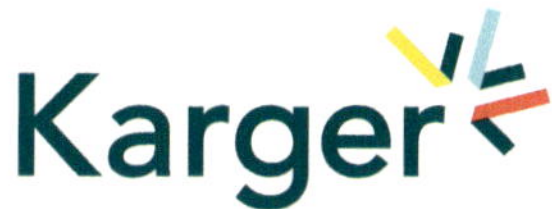

HEALTHCARE

What is alpha thalassemia?

Thalassemia is a condition you are born with. It affects **red blood cells**. There are two main types: alpha thalassemia (AT) and beta thalassemia (BT). This booklet is about AT.

In AT, the body doesn't make enough healthy **hemoglobin** (Hb) and there are too few red blood cells. Hb is the protein in red blood cells that enables them to carry oxygen around the body.

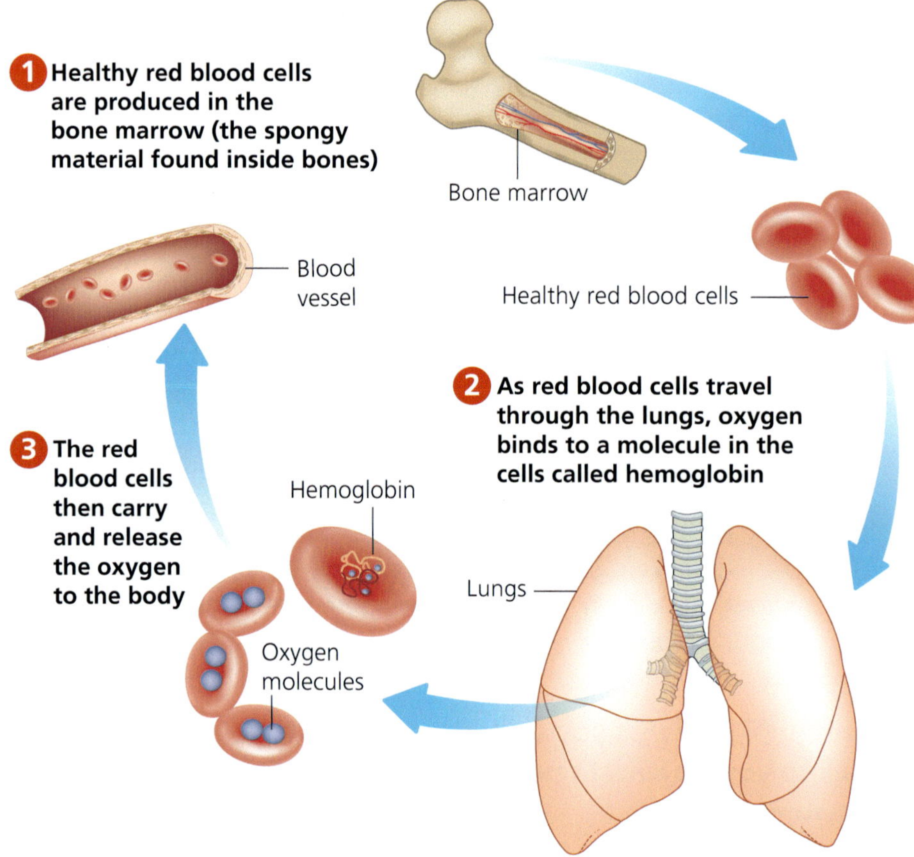

Why isn't the hemoglobin made properly?

Hb is the protein molecule in red blood cells that carries oxygen from the lungs to the tissues of the body. Carbon dioxide is also transported by Hb from the tissues back to the lungs. Hb helps maintain the shape of a red blood cell.

Normal adult Hb is made up of four protein chains – two alpha chains and two beta chains. If you have AT, your body either makes abnormal alpha chains or doesn't produce enough of them, so you can't make enough healthy Hb.

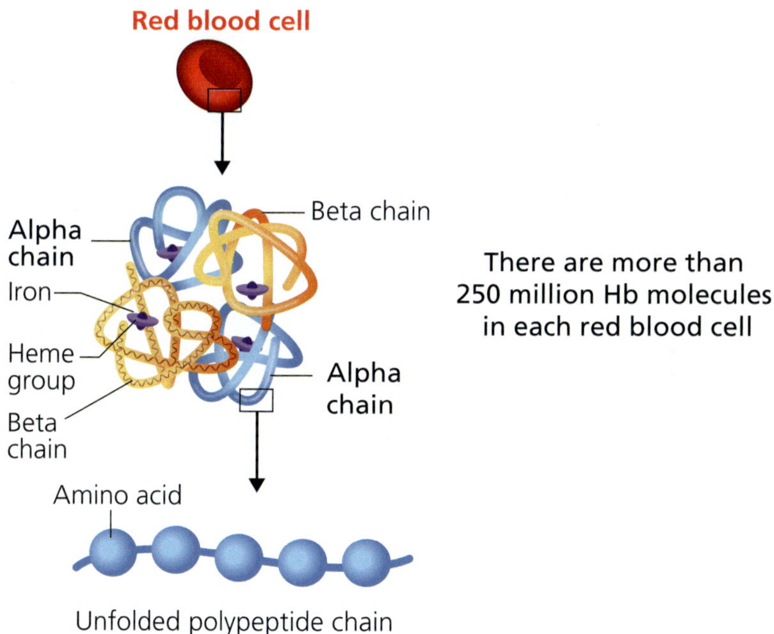

There are more than 250 million Hb molecules in each red blood cell

When there aren't enough healthy red blood cells and Hb, oxygen does not reach the tissues of the body, and a person can feel weak, tired and have difficulty breathing. This is called **anemia**. It can be mild or serious. Serious anemia can damage organs and can be fatal.

What causes AT and who gets it?

AT is a **genetic condition**. This means it is caused by a change (**mutation**) in one or more **genes**. There can be different types of change – some cause the alpha chains of Hb to be missing completely, while others cause a decrease in alpha chain production.

AT is more common in some parts of the world where malaria is, or has been, a problem (for example, the Middle East, northern Africa, India and Southeast Asia) and in people with ancestry originating from these areas. This is because the gene changes that cause AT also give some protection against malaria.

Over time, the proportion of people in the population with an AT gene change has increased and, as people migrate around the world, AT has become more common in other regions too.

My questions

Note down any questions that you have about how AT is caused to discuss with your doctor

Types of AT

The type of AT you have and how it affects you depends on:
- how many genes are changed and which ones
- the combination of genes that are affected
- whether each affected gene is completely missing or damaged.

Four types of AT

Silent carrier. Blood tests are usually normal. You will often have no symptoms, but you can pass the damaged gene on to your child.

Alpha thalassemia minor/trait. You may have mild anemia with small red blood cells that may be mistaken for iron deficiency anemia. Two genes are affected.

Hemoglobin H (HbH) AT. There is just one working alpha gene. You may have moderate to severe anemia. You have a greater risk of having a child with AT major.

Alpha thalassemia major. All four genes are missing. This causes severe anemia. In most cases, a baby with this condition will die before birth unless they are treated in the womb.

You can read more about genes and genetic inheritance on page 6.

My type of AT

Ask your doctor what type of AT you have.
Note it down here

Read more about gene changes on page 7.

Genes and genetic inheritance

Genes are carried on **chromosomes**. Every cell in our bodies has 23 pairs of chromosomes – so 46 in total. Every chromosome carries anywhere from 55 to 20 000 genes.

Genes are in pairs too. You inherit one copy from your mother and one copy from your father. A pair of genes is carried on a pair of chromosomes (one gene on each chromosome). Each pair of genes carries the code to make a single protein. Proteins are chains of chemical building blocks called **amino acids** and they are vital for the body to function.

Altogether, your genes carry the blueprint for the growth, development and function of your entire body.

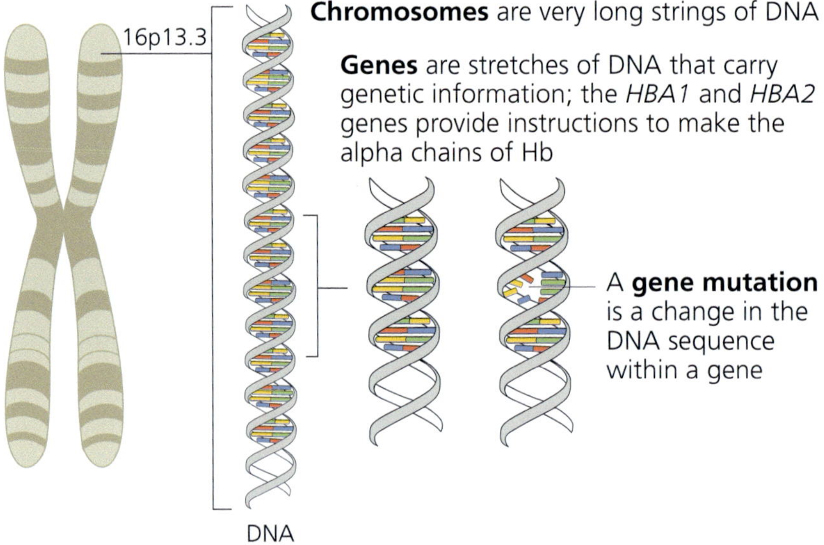

Which genes are involved?

Production of the Hb alpha chains is controlled by two pairs of genes – *HBA1* and *HBA2*. The codes they carry are the same.

Each person inherits one copy of each gene from their father and another copy of each gene from their mother. This means that there are four gene copies that can potentially cause AT:

- Two *HBA1* genes
- Two *HBA2* genes.

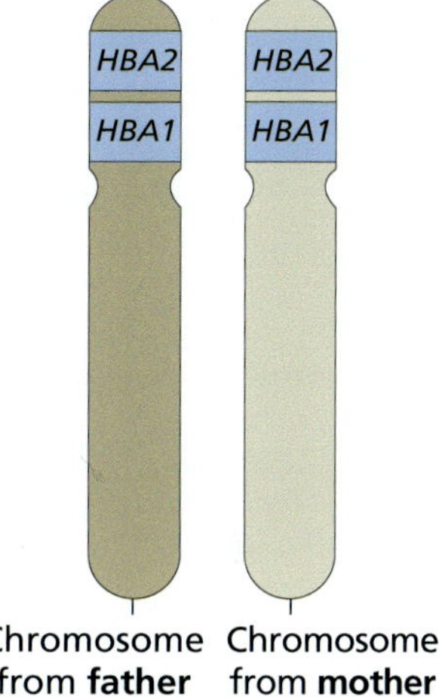

Deletional and non-deletional gene changes. There are two important types of gene change in AT.

- If a gene is completely missing, it is called **deletional thalassemia**.
- If a gene is not missing but is damaged, it is called **non-deletional thalassemia**. Non-deletional gene changes tend to cause more severe symptoms than deletional ones.

Location of gene changes. If you have two gene changes, the missing or damaged genes can both be on the same chromosome. This is called a 'cis' mutation (gene change). You may see this written as aa/-- in your notes.

Or there may be one gene change on each chromosome. This is called a 'trans' mutation. You may see this written as a-/a- in your notes.

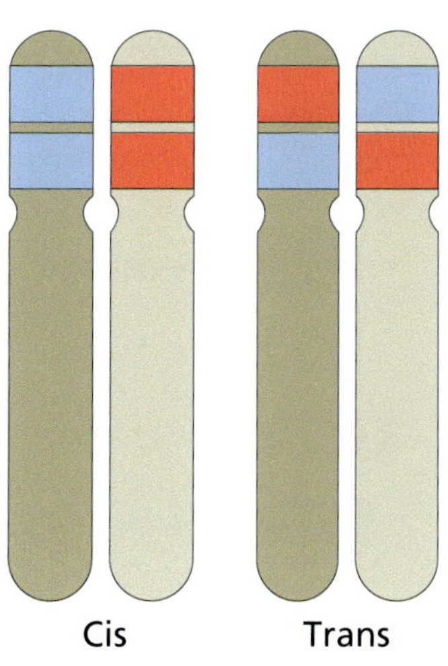

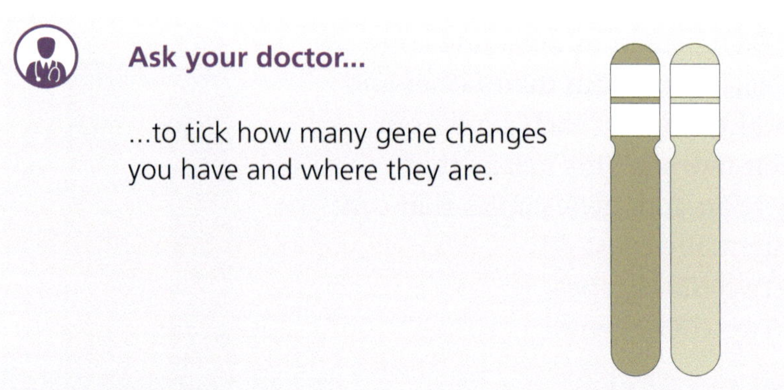

Ask your doctor...

...to tick how many gene changes you have and where they are.

Why is it important to know more about my condition?

If you are pregnant or planning to become pregnant, it is important to understand more about your genetic condition. Understanding more means you are better informed about the risks to your unborn child.

It is important for parents to know if the gene changes are on the same chromosome or on different chromosomes.

Ask your doctor about your gene changes and write the information in the box at the top of this page.

The following pages explain in more detail the different changes and what they may mean for you and your family.

One gene change	Turn to	**Page 9**
Two gene changes	Turn to	**Page 10**
Three gene changes	Turn to	**Page 14**
Four gene changes	Turn to	**Page 20**

One gene change

If you have only one AT gene change, you are said to be a **silent carrier**. This is also called **AT minima**.

What does this mean?

You won't have any signs of AT and will have no health problems related to it.

If you are a carrier and you have a child with someone who is also a carrier, for each pregnancy there is a:

- 1 in 4 chance (25%) the baby will have AT trait (two gene changes, see page 9)
- 1 in 2 chance (50%) the baby will be a silent carrier (one gene change)
- 1 in 4 chance (25%) the baby won't have any gene changes.

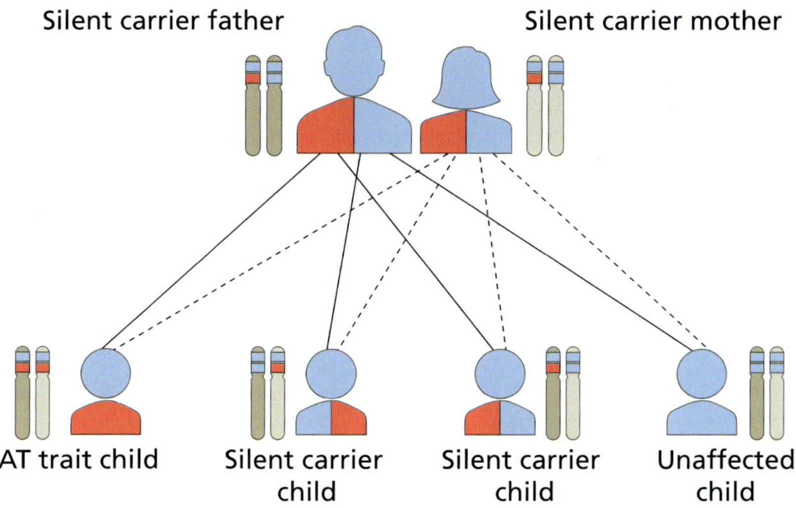

Very rarely, and only with certain kinds of gene change, there is a chance of having a child with AT.

Two gene changes

If you have two gene changes, you are said to have **AT trait**, which is also called **AT minor**.

What does this mean?

Most people with two gene changes don't have any serious health problems related to AT, apart from mild **anemia** (a shortage of healthy red blood cells). Anemia can cause fatigue, particularly after exercise (see page 29).

Under a microscope, your red blood cells will look smaller than usual. Doctors call small red blood cells **microcytosis**. The cells look like this because of a lack of Hb.

IMPORTANT: If you're anemic, make sure your doctor knows that you have AT trait (or that there is thalassemia in your family if you haven't been tested). If the doctor doesn't know this, they may prescribe an iron supplement for your anemia but that's something you definitely don't need if you have AT because you may develop 'iron overload'. Iron overload is harmful (see page 33).

Commonly used words

Microcytosis is the term used to describe red blood cells that are unusually small.

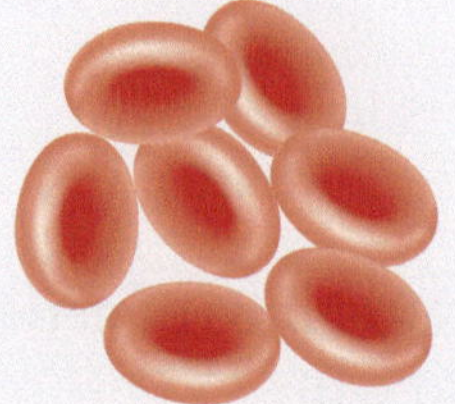

Normal red blood cells

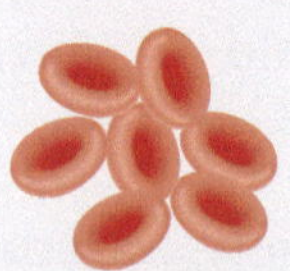

Microcytic red blood cells

When **one parent has two gene changes on the same chromosome and the other parent has no gene changes**, for each pregnancy there is a:

- 1 in 2 chance (50%) the baby will have AT trait (two gene changes)
- 1 in 2 chance (50%) the baby won't have any gene changes.

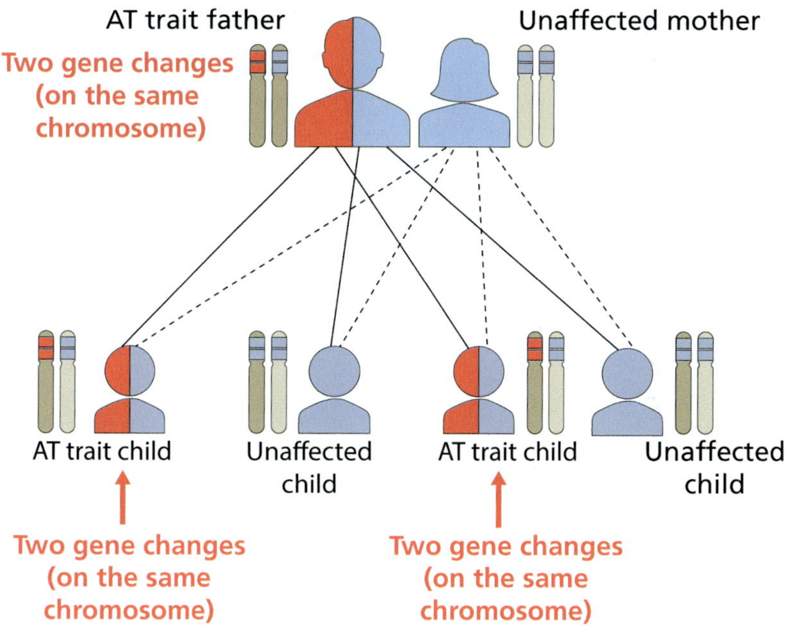

If both parents have two gene changes on the same chromosome, for each pregnancy there is a:

- 1 in 4 chance (25%) the baby will have AT major (four gene changes)
- 1 in 2 chance (50%) the baby will have AT trait with two gene changes on the same chromosome
- 1 in 4 chance (25%) the baby won't have any gene changes.

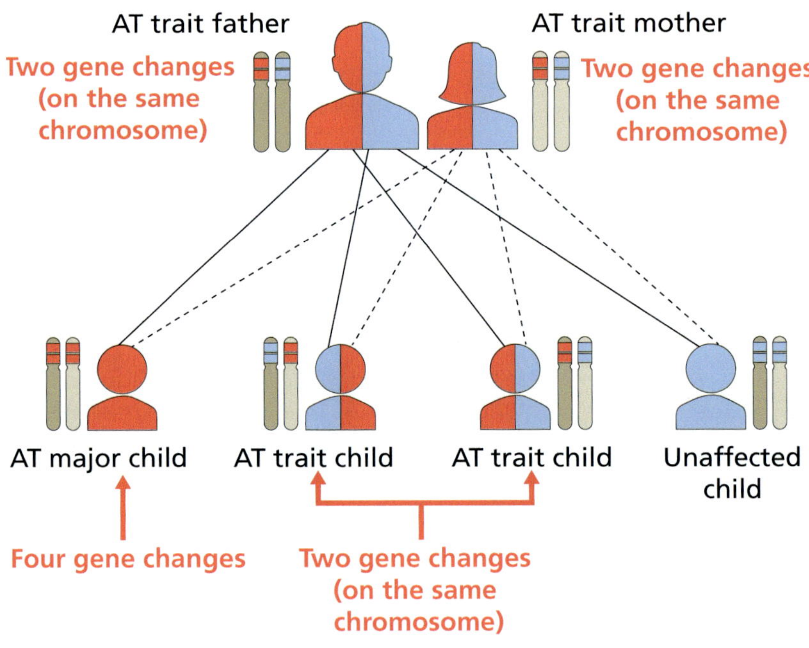

If one parent has gene changes on each chromosome but the other parent has no gene changes, every child will be a carrier.

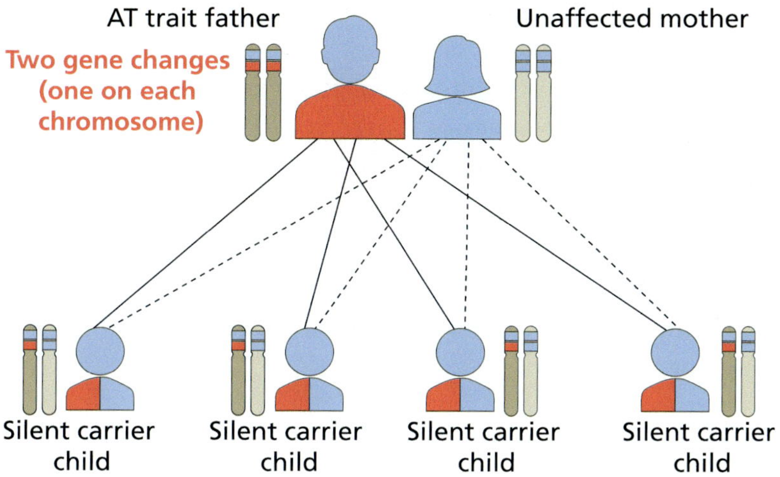

If both parents have gene changes on each chromosome, every child will have AT trait.

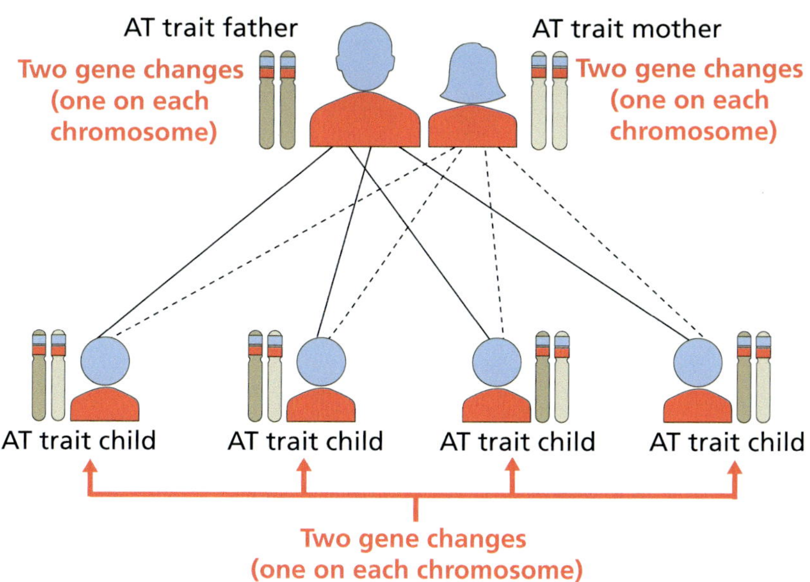

Three gene changes

If you have three gene changes, you have **Hemoglobin H AT (HbH AT)**.

What does this mean?

The symptoms and complications you experience will depend on the type of gene change you have.

People with **non-deletional HbH** tend to have more severe disease than people with missing AT genes (**deletional HbH**).

You may have only mild anemia or it may be severe enough for you to need regular **blood transfusions** from a young age.

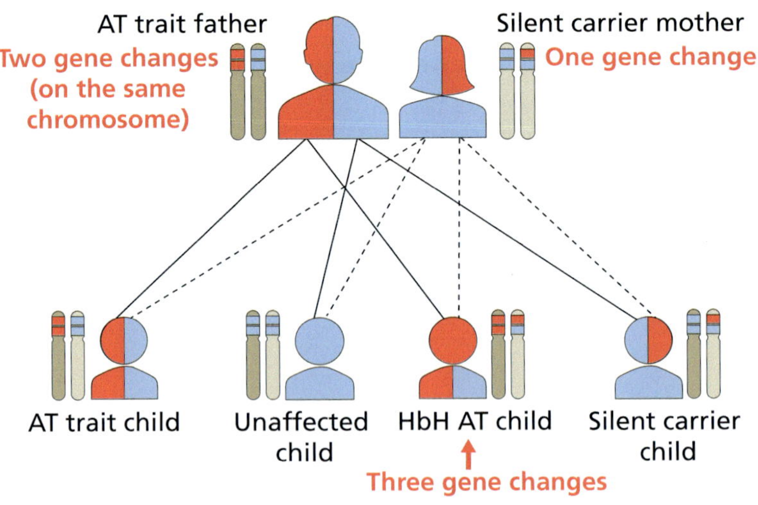

What is the risk if I have children?

If one parent has three gene changes but the other parent has no changes, for each pregnancy there is a:

- 1 in 2 chance (50%) the baby will be a carrier (one gene change)
- 1 in 2 chance (50%) the baby will have AT trait (two gene changes on the same chromosome).

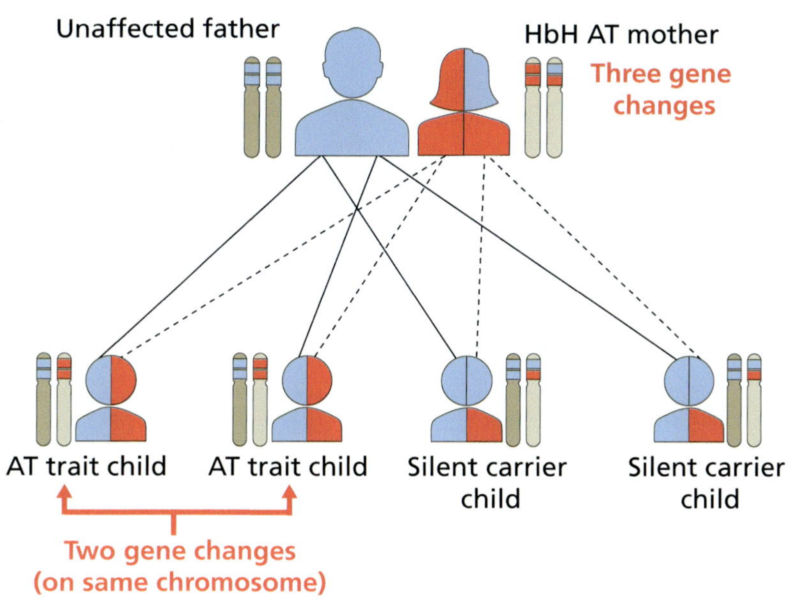

If one parent has three gene changes and the other has one gene change, for each pregnancy there is a:

- 1 in 4 chance (25%) the baby will be a carrier (one gene change)
- 1 in 2 chance (50%) the baby will have AT trait (two gene changes)
- 1 in 4 chance (25%) the baby will have HbH AT (three gene changes).

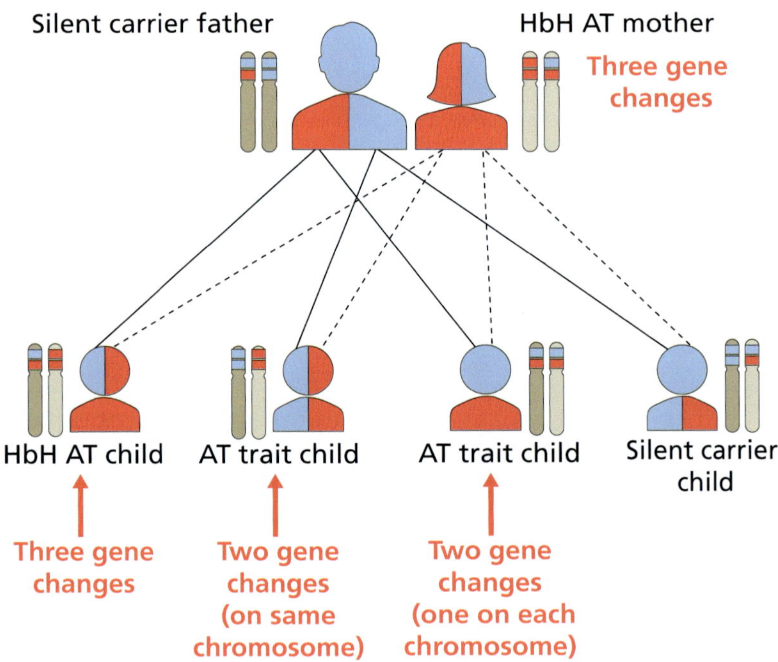

If one parent has three gene changes and the other has two gene changes on the same chromosome, for each pregnancy there is a:

- 1 in 4 chance (25%) the baby will be a carrier (one gene change)
- 1 in 4 chance (25%) the baby will have AT trait (two gene changes on the same chromosome)
- 1 in 4 chance (25%) the baby will have HbH AT (three gene changes)
- 1 in 4 chance (25%) the baby will have AT major (four gene changes).

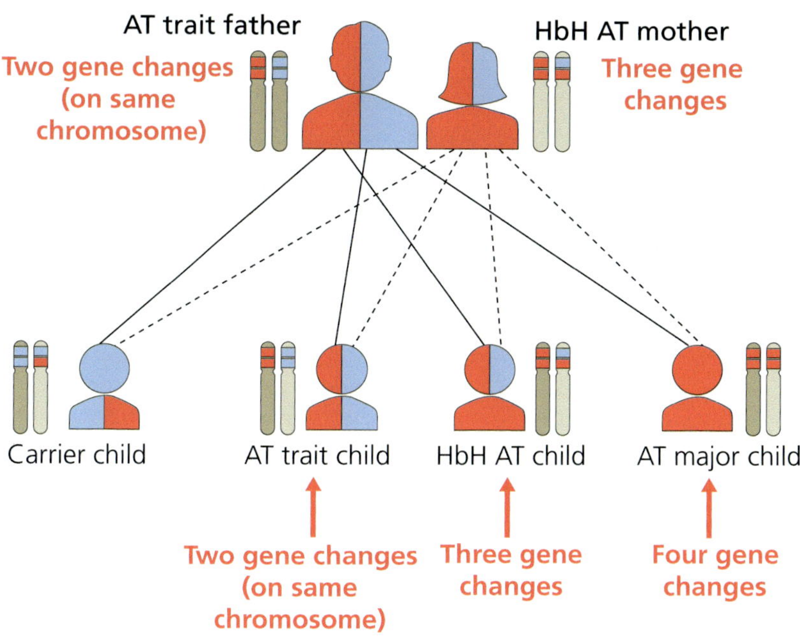

If one parent has three gene changes and the other has two gene changes, one on each chromosome, for each pregnancy there is a:

- 1 in 2 chance (50%) the baby will have AT trait (two gene changes changes, one on each chromosome)
- 1 in 2 chance (50%) the baby will have HbH AT (three gene changes).

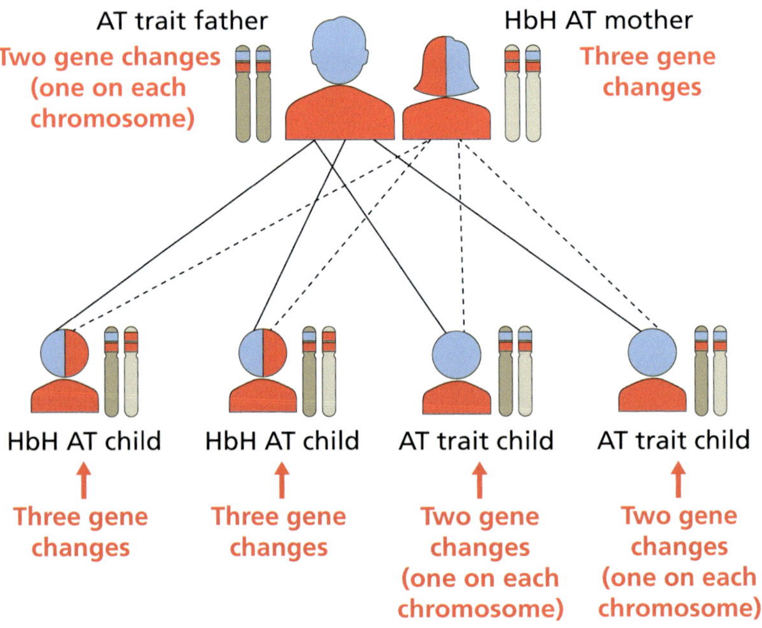

If both parents have three gene changes, for each pregnancy there is a:

- 1 in 4 chance (25%) the baby will have AT trait (two gene changes on the same chromosome)
- 1 in 2 chance (50%) the baby will have HbH AT (three gene changes)
- 1 in 4 chance (25%) the baby will have AT major (four gene changes).

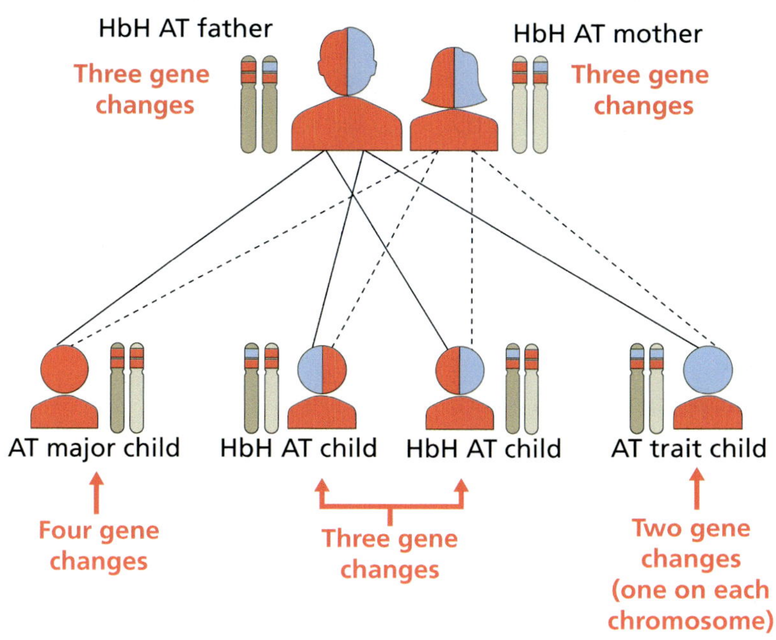

Four gene changes

If you have four gene changes, you have no genes that make alpha chains properly. This is called **AT major** or **Hb Barts disease**. This is the most serious form of AT.

What does this mean?

When a baby starts to develop in the womb, the first type of Hb its body makes is called **embryonic Hb**, which doesn't include any alpha chains. By 16 weeks, the baby begins to make another type of Hb called **fetal Hb**, which needs alpha chains.

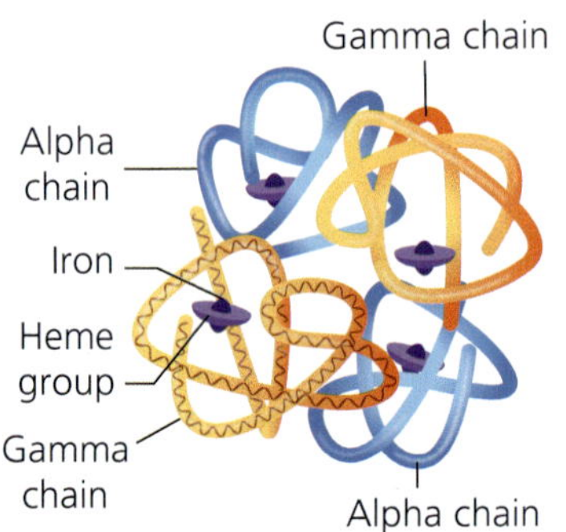

Fetal Hb is made up of alpha and gamma Hb chains; if no alpha chains can be made, four gamma chains form an abnormal type of Hb called Hb Barts

A baby with four gene changes can't make alpha chains, so fetal Hb cannot develop. Instead, a type of Hb called Hb Barts is made. The baby will develop severe anemia and will die in the womb without treatment. Doctors call this '**hydrops fetalis**' (or just 'hydrops' for short).

It may be possible for the baby to have red blood cell transfusions while still inside the womb (this is called **intrauterine transfusion**), so the chance of the baby living until birth is greatly increased. However, there is still a high risk of premature birth.

Your health will also be closely monitored throughout your pregnancy. Your medical team will do everything they can to lower the risk of complications for both you and the baby.

What is the risk if I have children?

If one parent has four gene changes and their partner has two gene changes on the same chromosome, for each pregnancy there is a:

- 1 in 2 chance (50%) the baby will have AT major (four gene changes)
- 1 in 2 chance (50%) the baby will have AT trait (two AT genes on the same chromosome).

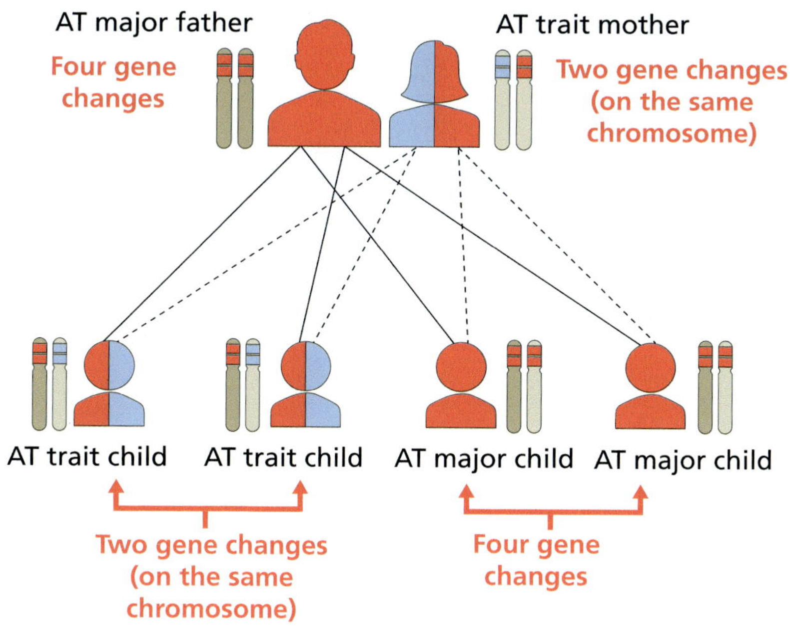

If one parent has four gene changes and their partner has two gene changes on different chromosomes, every child will have HbH AT (three gene changes).

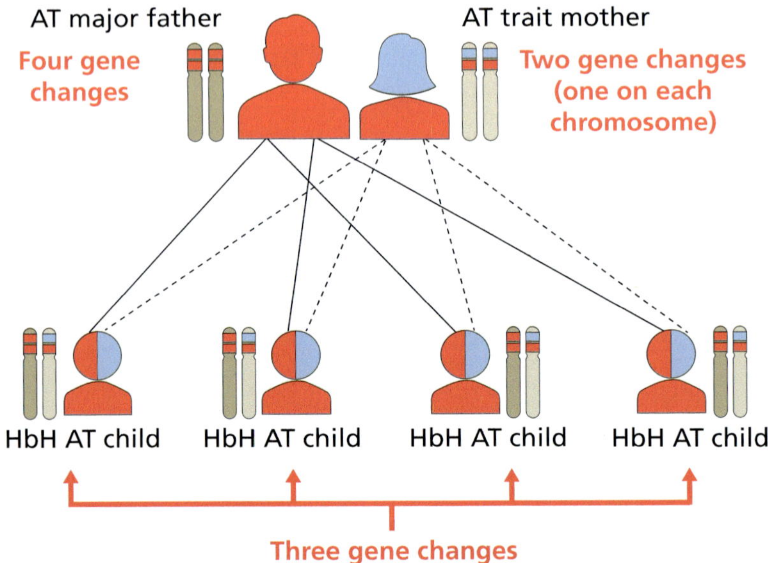

If one parent has four gene changes and their partner has HbH AT (three gene changes), for each pregnancy there is a:
- 1 in 2 chance (50%) the baby will have AT major (four gene changes)
- 1 in 2 chance (50%) the baby will have HbH AT (three gene changes).

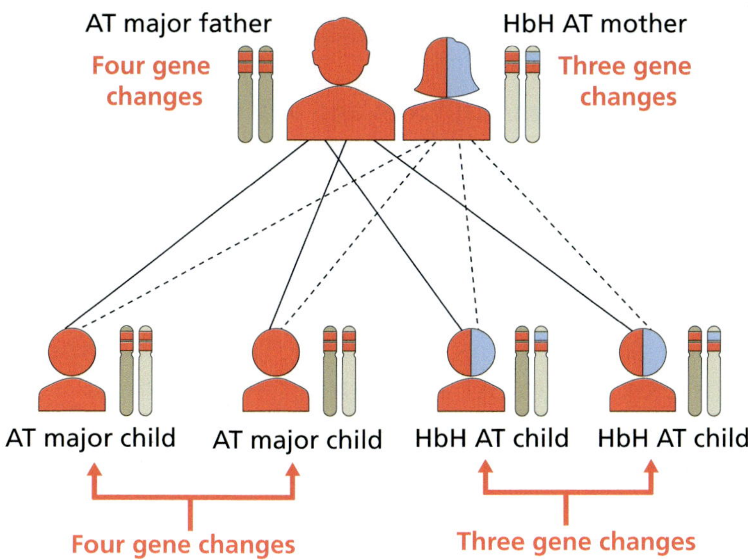

Screening and diagnosis

Newborn screening

In some parts of the world, all newborn babies have a blood test for thalassemia. A nurse pricks the baby's heel with a fine needle and squeezes out a drop of blood. This is used to test for other genetic conditions as well.

It is unlikely that the test will find one or two gene changes but it is likely to find HbH AT (three gene changes) (see page 14).

Diagnostic testing in children and adults

A doctor may suggest testing for thalassemia because you (or your child) show some of the symptoms of AT or if a routine blood test shows that you or your child have mild microcytic anemia.

Often, doctors test for iron deficiency first because it's a common cause of microcytic anemia. They will do other tests to look for HbH AT and AT trait (see page 29).

These tests can't show how many AT genes are affected though.

To identify the exact genetic changes, you'll need to have DNA tests done on a blood sample.

My concerns and questions

Note down any questions that you have about your AT for discussion with your doctor

Genetic counseling

Before having screening tests for thalassemia, you may be offered **genetic counseling**. This is to make sure you understand any tests you might have and what the results may mean.

Usually, the partners of people with two gene changes on the same chromosome or three gene changes (HbH AT) will also need to have a DNA test.

The counselor will continue to provide support after testing if results show that there is a risk that your children could have three or four gene changes. You will be able to discuss the options when planning a pregnancy.

Some couples decide to have **in vitro fertilization** (also known as IVF or a 'test-tube baby') so that genetic testing can be carried out before the fertilized egg is implanted in the womb. Depending on the gene changes that the parents have, genetic testing can make sure that the baby doesn't have AT major (see page 20) or doesn't have any AT gene changes at all.

Pregnancy screening

If you're already pregnant, your doctor will want to do genetic testing early in the pregnancy in case your baby needs treatment before birth. This helps to prevent premature birth and avoid serious complications for the mother.

If there is a risk that the baby could have AT major, the doctor will suggest testing the baby while still in the womb.

There are different ways to do the test:

- taking a sample of blood from the umbilical cord (**cordocentesis**)
- testing the fluid surrounding the baby (**amniocentesis**)
- taking a sample of the placenta (**chorionic villus sampling**).

Which test you have depends on how far through the pregnancy you are. All the tests carry a small risk of miscarriage, so your doctor will only suggest testing if it is absolutely necessary.

Ultrasound analysis may be used and some non-invasive tests are currently under investigation, such as testing fetal DNA found in the mother's bloodstream. These may be useful in future, but they are currently not accurate enough to use for thalassemia and give high levels of wrong results.

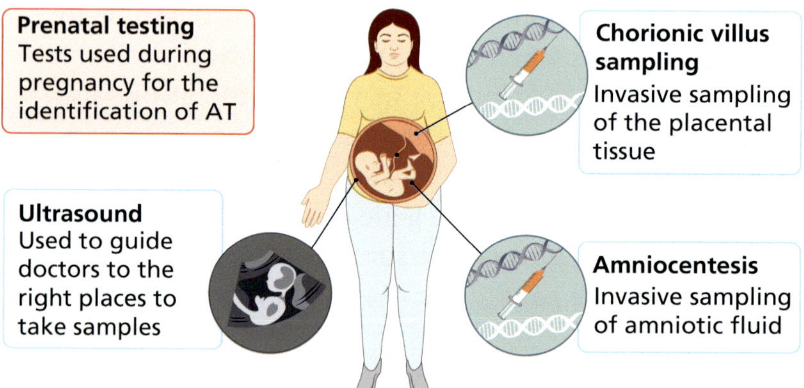

Commonly used words

Invasive sampling means a sample of tissue or fluid is taken from inside the body. This is done via a cut in the skin or through a body opening.

Babies and AT major. Birth defects are more likely in babies born with AT major, even if they have blood transfusions in the womb. The most common birth defects are minor abnormalities of the genitals in boys. For example, the opening of the urethra (the tube you pee through) can be on the underside of the penis. This is called hypospadias and can be fixed with surgery.

Around 1 in 6 babies (about 17%) have a limb abnormality. These vary in how severe they are. Examples include having hands of different sizes or part of a foot that hasn't fully developed.

A baby with **AT major** (see page 20) who does not receive an intrauterine transfusion before he is born will be likely to die in the womb.

Depending on the results of the tests, your counselor may take you through the difficult decision of whether to continue with the pregnancy. There is no single answer that suits every couple. The decision depends on many factors, including cultural, social, spiritual and religious beliefs.

Pregnancy

A pregnant woman with AT needs special care during her pregnancy. Anemia can become more severe (see page 29). A condition called **pre-eclampsia** is also more common, which can be fatal if not detected. Signs of pre-eclampsia include rising blood pressure and protein in the urine (signs of damage to the liver or kidneys).

The mother will have regular tests for these during her pregnancy and will often take medication to lower blood pressure.

Symptoms and treatment
How will AT affect me or my child?

Symptoms of AT vary depending on which type of AT you have. Some people have no symptoms while others have severe symptoms that need lifelong treatment.

Complications are health problems caused by the disease (AT) or by the treatment. Complications also vary from mild to severe.

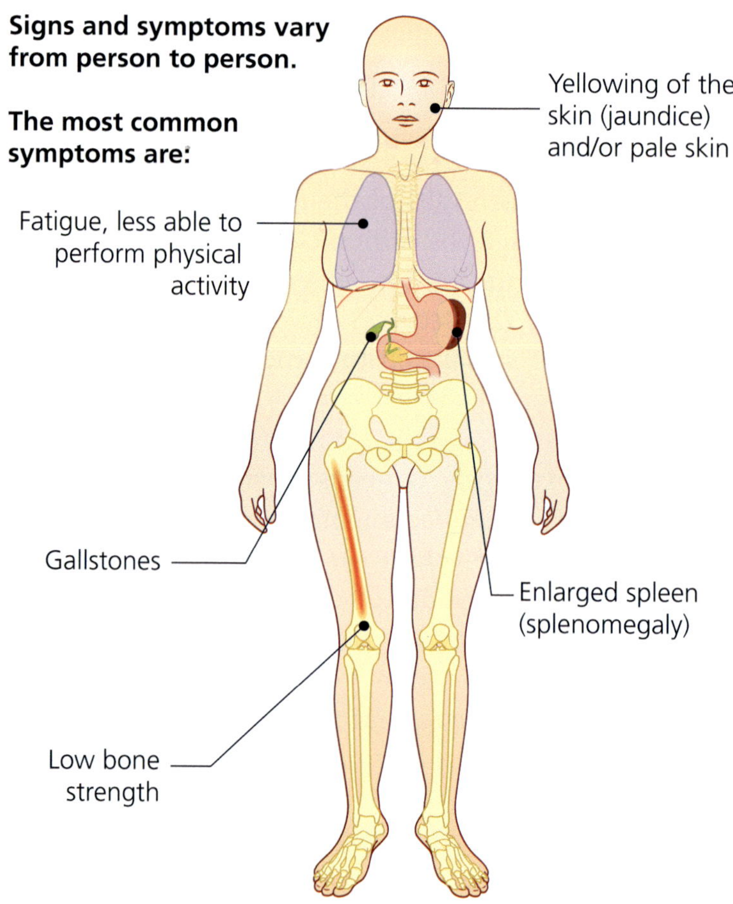

Silent carrier (page 9). As a silent carrier, you won't have any symptoms of AT and will have no health problems related to AT.

AT trait (page 10). With AT trait, symptoms vary from none to **mild anemia**. This can cause fatigue, particularly after exercise, and pale skin and you may feel weak.

HbH AT (page 14). Symptoms and complications are more severe in people with HbH AT. They include anemia, enlarged liver and spleen, gallstones, abnormal bone development, blood clots and iron overload (see below).

AT major (page 20). Children and adults with AT major will need regular treatment to prevent severe anemia. They are also at risk of all the complications that can happen with HbH AT (see below).

Anemia

People with more severe HbH AT and AT major will have more severe anemia, which causes increased fatigue, difficulty breathing, weakness and dizziness.

Anemia can sometimes get worse with age or when the body is under stress: for example, if you have an infection or during pregnancy.

Babies born with HbH AT may have anemia but don't usually need regular treatment.

Children and adults with AT major will need regular treatment for anemia.

Treatment. The main treatment for anemia is **blood transfusions**. Blood transfusions provide healthy red blood cells.

How often will I need blood transfusions? How often people with HbH AT (three gene changes) need blood transfusions varies. It depends on how severe their anemia is and it also depends on their age. Some people with HbH AT need regular transfusions by

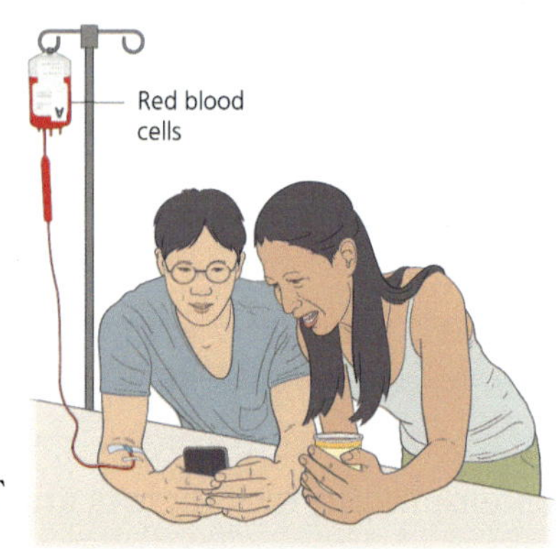

the time they reach their teens or 20s.

People with **AT major** (four gene changes; see page 20) will need regular transfusions throughout their lives. Transfusions can happen every couple of weeks.

You receive blood through a small plastic tube inserted into one of the blood vessels in your arm. The procedure usually happens in a hospital or a special clinic for blood diseases. Babies, children and adults can have transfusions. The procedure will take a few hours each time.

Doctors also sometimes prescribe folic acid tablets to help with anemia. Folic acid is a kind of vitamin which helps to produce red blood cells.

Enlarged liver and spleen

HbH AT and AT major can cause the liver and spleen
to get bigger than normal, and your abdomen may feel
uncomfortable. You may have pain too. It happens because
the spleen has to work hard to get rid of the faulty red blood
cells and the liver has to work hard to process the resulting
waste products.

Treatment. If an enlarged spleen is causing discomfort
and pain, you may need surgery to remove it. The removal
of a spleen is called **splenectomy**. Blood transfusions can
also help to shrink an enlarged spleen. People who have
had a splenectomy have a higher risk of infections. Your
hematologist and general surgeon will discuss the risks and
benefits with you.

Gallstones

These can develop because of high levels of bilirubin
(a waste product from the processing of red blood cells).
Some people with gallstones have no symptoms, but others
may feel bloated and sick (nauseated) and have abdomen pain.

Treatment. The treatment is usually laparoscopic surgery
(sometimes called keyhole or bandaid surgery) to remove
your gallbladder. Keyhole surgery usually means that you
recover more quickly because there is no major incision.

Abnormal bone development

Normally, blood cells are made inside the bones by a tissue called **bone marrow**. In AT there are fewer circulating red blood cells and less Hb than normal. To try to make up for this, the bone marrow becomes overactive and produces more and more red blood cells. But as these are abnormal, they die early and don't help to correct the anemia. As the bone marrow continues to try to correct the anemia, it expands and this may cause the bones to become bigger, particularly in the face, causing a 'heavy' forehead and overgrowth of the brows and jaw. Your doctor may call this **bossing**.

With untreated AT, limbs can also be shorter than usual because the long bones stop growing early. Bones may also become weakened and break more easily. Your doctor may call this **osteoporosis** or **osteopenia**.

Treatment. If you or your child have HbH AT or AT major, you will have regular health checks so that any abnormal bone development is found early. Regular blood transfusions and the treatment for iron overload usually helps prevent bone problems (see pages 34 and 35).

Blood clots

People with AT have a slightly increased risk of blood clots. The risk is higher in people who have had their spleen removed and the risk increases with age. Blood clots are more common in women.

Treatment. Treatment for blood clots varies but may include aspirin or low-dose blood thinners. These are called **anticoagulants**.

Leg ulcers

HbH AT can cause problems with wound healing. Even minor wounds on the legs, particularly the ankles, don't heal and may become infected and need antibiotics.

Iron overload

Iron overload is a common complication of AT major and HbH AT.

Normally, when aging red blood cells are broken down in the body, the iron that's released is recycled into new cells. When a person has regular blood transfusions, iron overload can happen as donor blood also contains iron. Iron overload is when there is too much iron in your body. It can also develop in people with HbH AT who do not have regular transfusions but it happens more slowly. The buildup occurs because the overactive bone marrow sends signals to the gut to absorb much more iron from the diet. This happens because the body tries to correct the anemia by making more red blood cells and for this it needs iron.

Why is iron overload a problem? Too much iron is toxic to the body as the body is not able to remove it. The excess iron increases over time and can damage your organs.

Iron buildup can damage the liver. The damaged liver tissue is replaced by fibrous tissue, also called scar tissue. This process is called **fibrosis**. A research study found that around 1 in 5 people (20%) with HbH AT have liver tissue that has been replaced with fibrous tissue (fibrosis).* If fibrosis gets worse, it can develop into liver cirrhosis and liver failure.

---

*Chan LKL, Mak VWM, Chan SCH et al. Liver complications of haemoglobin H disease in adults. *British Journal of Haematology* 2020;192:171–8.

Iron overload can cause heart damage, leading to abnormal heart rhythms (arrhythmia) and eventually heart failure.

It can also damage your bones and joints. People with AT major and HbH AT are prone to weakened bones (osteoporosis). This is partly due to the thalassemia, but iron overload also contributes because iron can collect in the bones and cause damage.

Hormone levels can be affected by iron overload. Your thyroid hormone levels may be low, leading to fatigue, weight gain and constipation. You may also be more at risk of developing diabetes, because iron affects the production of insulin in the pancreas, which controls your blood sugar levels.

If you are receiving blood transfusions, you may have low levels of sex hormones. In children with AT, this can mean that puberty is later than usual. This is less common these days, because many children have well-managed anemia and iron levels after their AT diagnosis.

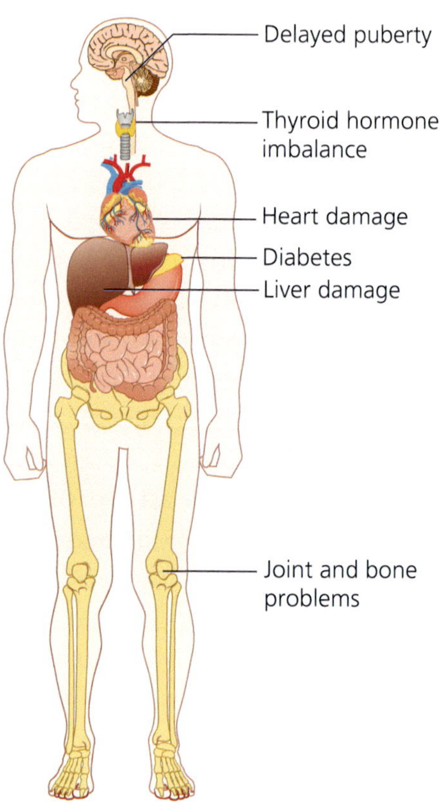

Iron overload can affect the body in a variety of ways

Treatment. To help prevent all the problems caused by iron toxicity, your iron levels may need to be controlled by a treatment called **chelation therapy**. There are three types of chelation therapy. You may have it through continuous intravenous infusion (directly into a vein), through your skin (subcutaneously) or by mouth (orally). Your doctor will discuss the choice of chelation therapy with you and any possible side effects.

Your doctor will monitor your iron level with blood tests. If it seems high, you may have an MRI (magnetic resonance imaging) scan to measure the iron concentration in your liver and/or your heart. This will show whether you need chelation therapy.

IMPORTANT: If your doctor says you need chelation therapy, it is very important that you follow their instructions. Iron overload can be fatal.

Your healthcare team

AT is a complex health condition and needs specialist care. Your treatment should be managed by a specialist center for blood disorders and overseen by a consultant **hematologist** (a doctor that specializes in treating blood disorders and diseases).

Specialist centers will often have a thalassemia clinical nurse specialist, who you can contact if you have any questions when you're at home.

Clinical trials

If you are interested in new treatments, you may want to ask your doctor about clinical trials. All new medical treatments have to be tested in clinical trials. A new treatment must go through several phases of testing before it can be proven to work better than existing treatment and be adopted into routine care. A potential treatment will only move on to the next phase of research if it is safe and shows promise.

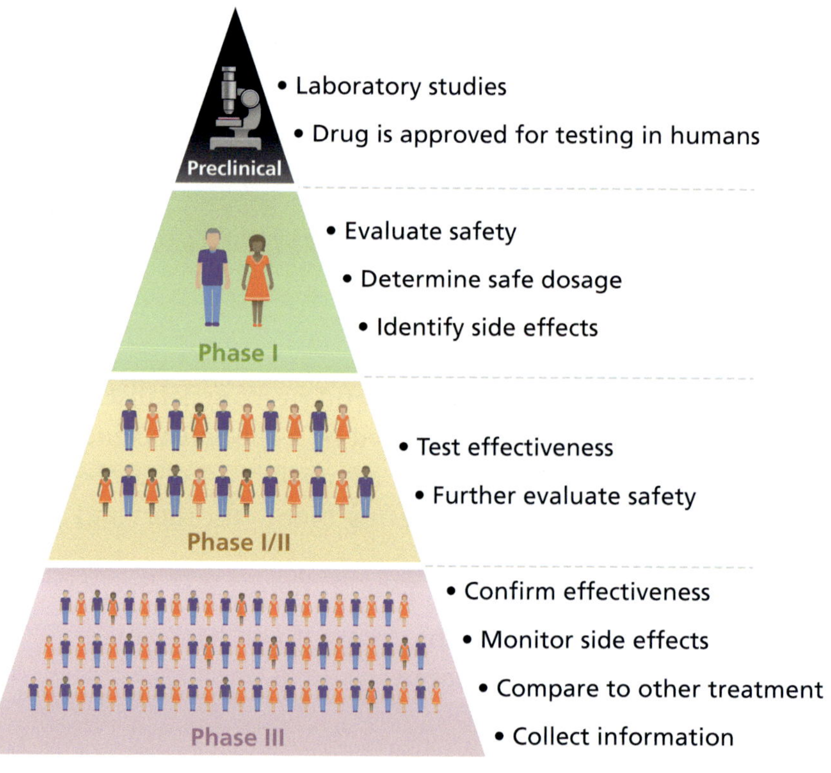

New treatments for AT
Slowing the breakdown of red blood cells

There has been some research looking into treating anemia in people with AT with medication to reduce the destruction of red blood cells.

Mitapivat is a new treatment that is being tested in people with AT or beta thalassemia. It's a tablet that you take twice a day. It's already used to treat another genetic condition that causes anemia, called pyruvate kinase deficiency.

This treatment helps to activate an enzyme that is needed for red blood cells to function properly. Early trial results show that it may be able to reduce anemia in people with AT who don't need regular blood transfusions. Side effects found so far include difficulty sleeping, headache and dizziness.

Mitapivat is being tested in a Phase III trial for people with AT who do and do not require regular transfusions.

Stem cell transplant

The only way to potentially cure AT is with a stem cell transplant from a donor. Stem cell transplant is currently only suitable for AT major, as the treatment itself has many side effects, some of which can be life-threatening.

Stem cells are cells in the bone marrow that can develop into all the different types of blood cell in the body, including red blood cells.

When you have a transplant, the stem cells in your bone marrow are destroyed and replaced with healthy cells from the donor. The donor must be someone whose blood cells closely match yours, and this is usually a close family member.

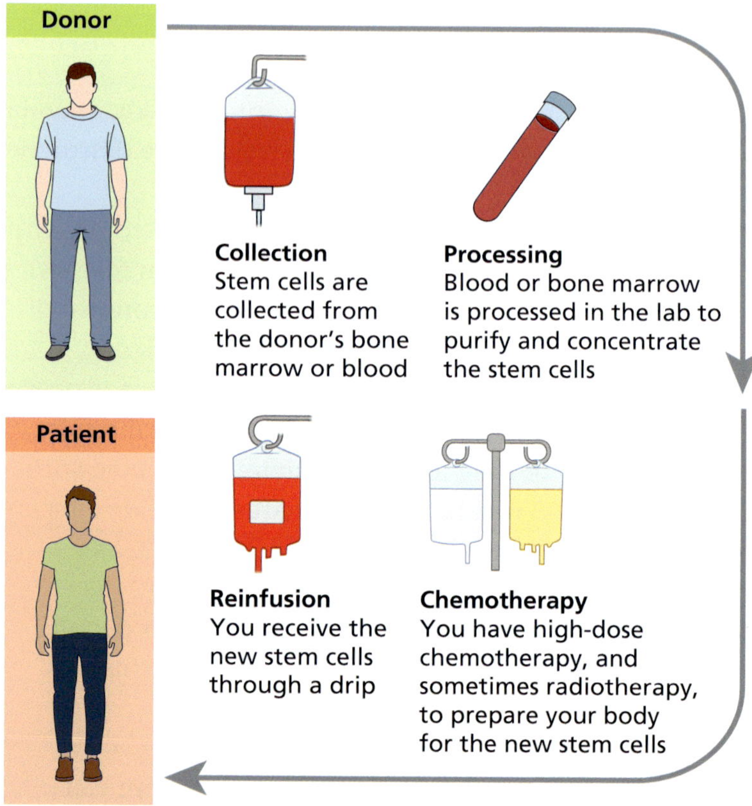

The aim is for the donor stem cells to start to grow inside your bones and provide new blood stem cells to replace yours. This process is called 'engraftment'. The new stem cells will produce all the different types of blood cells, including healthy red blood cells.

Until the new stem cells have started to work, you have a very high risk of infection. So, you need to be nursed in isolation for some time after having your stem cell infusion.

Living with alpha thalassemia

Some people with AT already know that it runs in their family. For others, it's a complete shock when they are diagnosed with AT because of anemia symptoms or when a baby is diagnosed shortly after birth. Genetic counseling can help you to understand your condition and its implications, including the risk to any future children you may have.

You are likely to have a lot of questions. It's important to find out as much as you can about AT and about your own situation.

AT is complicated and it's easy to get confused. It may help to write down a list of the things you need to know or questions you want to ask and take it to your doctor's appointment. It may also help to take someone with you, so you can compare notes afterwards.

Should I tell other people?

When should you tell people that you are a thalassemia carrier or have AT trait? The simple answer is: whenever you are ready. Mostly, you don't have to tell people if you don't want to. But you particularly need to be open with your partner if you are thinking of starting a family in the future. They will need to be tested too.

Talking about a genetic problem can be difficult. People sometimes feel it's their fault. But you have no control over the genes you inherit. You can use this booklet to help others understand more about AT.

IMPORTANT: Living a healthy life is important for everyone. When you have thalassemia, healthy choices are particularly important.

The best way to avoid complications is to stick to any treatment schedules and go to all your check-up appointments.

 **IMPORTANT:** Contact your doctor promptly if you have any signs of infection or other illness, and make sure you keep your vaccinations up to date – especially if you've had your spleen removed.

Your diet

It's important to look after your general health. Make sure you eat well.

People with thalassemia often have low levels of some vitamins and minerals, such as zinc. This is partly because of the anemia, and partly because of high iron levels and the treatment used to remove iron. Your doctor may give you supplements.

Some doctors suggest avoiding foods that contain iron, but others think that this has little effect in preventing iron overload. It's best to discuss your diet with your own AT healthcare team.

Keep fit for healthy bones

Regular physical exercise has many benefits. It can improve your mood and help strengthen your bones. Alcohol and smoking are best avoided.

Ask for help if you need to

Do ask questions and tell your healthcare team about anything that's concerning you. They know how complex AT is and won't mind, even if you ask the same questions more than once.

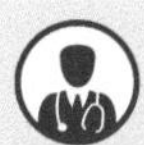

Questions for your doctor

What type of AT do I/does my child have?

How many gene changes are there?

Are they deletional or non-deletional gene changes?

What are the implications of the gene changes I have?

What impact will AT have on me/my child?

Will I/they need regular treatment?

What are the likely side effects of treatment?

What complications could there be and how likely are they?

What is the likelihood of me having another child with AT?

Is there anything that can be done to reduce the risk of having another child with AT?

Will my child with AT be able to have children and what do they need to know beforehand?

You can record the names and contact details of your doctors, nurses and other support staff here

Name   ....

Role   ....

Phone   ....

Email   ....

Name   ....

Role   ....

Phone   ....

Email   ....

Name   ....

Role   ....

Phone   ....

Email   ....

Guide to words and phrases

Alpha chain. A type of polypeptide chain needed to make normal adult hemoglobin. Can be missing or reduced in people with AT.

Anemia. A shortage of healthy red blood cells, which can cause symptoms of fatigue and breathlessness.

Anticoagulants. Medicines that reduce blood clotting.

AT major. All four genes that produce hemoglobin alpha chains are damaged or missing. Sometimes called Hb Barts disease.

AT minima. Now called 'silent carrier'; one of the four alpha chain genes is damaged or missing.

AT minor. Now called AT trait.

AT trait. Of the four genes that normally produce alpha chains, two are damaged or missing.

Bilirubin. A pigment produced when old and damaged red blood cells are destroyed.

Blood transfusion. Receiving donated blood through a drip (intravenous infusion) directly into your bloodstream.

Bone marrow. Spongy substance in the center of bones where blood cells are made.

Carrier. Term used to mean someone who carries and can pass on a gene change associated with a disease, but does not have the disease themselves.

Chelation therapy. Treatment used to remove excess metals from the body – in the case of AT this is iron.

Chromosomes. Long coiled strands of DNA. There are 23 pairs of chromosomes in human cells and one chromosome of each pair is inherited from each parent. Each chromosome carries many genes.

Cirrhosis. A liver disease caused by long-term liver damage. Healthy liver tissue is replaced with fibrous scar tissue and the liver shrinks.

Cis mutation. In AT trait, this means having two gene changes on the same chromosome.

Clinical trial. A research study to investigate a new test, treatment or medical procedure in people. Trials may look at whether a treatment is safe, its side effects or how well a treatment works.

Deletional. A deletional gene change in AT means the gene is completely missing.

DNA. The genetic code that is the blueprint for how an organism develops and functions. Genes and chromosomes are made of DNA.

Ferritin. A protein that stores iron inside your cells.

Fetal Hb. A type of hemoglobin that is only found in babies in the womb and for a short time after birth. After birth, adult hemoglobin is produced under the instructions of other genes.

Fibrosis. Thickening and stiffening of normal body tissues. Iron overload in AT can cause fibrosis of the liver.

Folic acid. A B vitamin necessary for red blood cell production. It is sometimes used to reduce anemia symptoms in people with AT.

Gallstones. Hard lumps that can form in your gallbladder and cause pain. In AT, they are caused by too much bilirubin (a by-product from the destruction of old or damaged red blood cells).

Gene. Stretches of DNA that carry the codes for individual proteins. They control growth and development of the body, and are grouped together to form chromosomes.

Genetic condition. A condition caused by a change in one or more genes.

Genetic counseling. A process that helps people come to terms with having a genetic condition running in their family and understand their risk of passing on that condition to a child.

Hb assessment. The blood test used to look at the types and amounts of hemoglobin present in a blood sample.

Hb Constant Spring (HbCS). A type of gene change found in AT that is named after the place where it was discovered.

Hb Barts disease. Another name for AT major.

HbH AT. Having three out of the four alpha chain genes missing or damaged. Symptoms are very variable between people and depend on the type of gene changes you have.

Hemoglobin. The iron-containing protein in red blood cells that binds to oxygen and carries it throughout the body.

Hemolysis. The breakdown of red blood cells and the release of their contents into the surrounding fluid (for example, the blood).

Hepatomegaly. An enlarged liver.

Hydrops fetalis. A serious condition that can develop in unborn babies with AT major. It causes abnormal collections of fluid in the body, which can be life-threatening.

Inheritance. Passing genes on to your children.

Intrauterine transfusion. A technique that enables a developing baby to have red blood cell transfusions while it is still in the womb.

Intravenous. Directly into a vein.

Iron-deficiency anemia. A type of anemia caused by a lack of iron. AT is not caused by lack of iron.

Iron overload. A complication of AT where too much iron builds up in the body and causes damage.

IVF. Stands for in vitro fertilization. Also known as 'test tube baby'. A woman's egg is fertilized outside the womb and then implanted back into it. Allows embryos to be screened for genetic conditions.

Jaundice. A yellowing of the skin and whites of the eyes caused by too much bilirubin in the body.

Laparoscopic surgery. The operation is carried out through several small incisions, so recovery is often quicker. Sometimes called keyhole surgery.

Liver. Body organ that processes waste products after hemolysis.

Malaria. A serious disease caused by a parasite transmitted to people by mosquitos. The disease is milder in people who carry the gene change for thalassemia.

Microcytosis. Means 'small cells'. People with AT trait may have unusually small red blood cells, which can be confused with iron deficiency anemia.

Mutation. A change in a gene.

Non-deletional. A gene change that means the gene is altered rather than missing, like a spelling error in the code.

Open surgery. Regular surgery, where the operation is carried out through a single large incision.

Osteopenia. Thinning of the bones that is not as severe as osteoporosis.

Osteoporosis. Thinning of the bones that weakens them and makes them prone to fracture.

Pre-eclampsia. A complication of pregnancy that can occur with hydrops fetalis. It can be fatal if not detected and treated. Signs in the mother include rising blood pressure and protein in the urine.

Protein. A type of molecule made up of at least one polypeptide chain (a chain of amino acids that are bound together) folded up into a three-dimensional shape.

Red blood cell. A type of blood cell that carries oxygen around the body.

Screening. Tests for a particular disease in people who do not have any symptoms.

'Silent carrier'. One AT gene change among the four genes that code for the hemoglobin alpha chain. You don't have the disease but can pass the gene change on to your children. Also called AT minima.

Spleen. Body organ that is part of the immune system and responsible for destroying old and damaged red blood cells.

Splenectomy. Surgery to remove the spleen.

Splenomegaly. An enlarged spleen.

Stem cell transplant. An intensive treatment for some types of blood disorders that is being researched as a potential cure for AT major.

Thrombosis. A blood clot.

Trait. (a) A genetic characteristic.
(b) Two gene changes in AT.

Trans mutation. In AT trait, this means that the two gene changes are on different chromosomes.

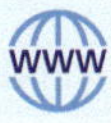

Recommended resources

Northern California Comprehensive Thalassemia Center
www.thalassemia.com

Thalassaemia International Federation
https://thalassaemia.org.cy

UK Thalassaemia Society
https://ukts.org

Cooley's Anemia Foundation
www.thalassemia.org

Sources used in the preparation of this document

BMJ Best Practice
https://bestpractice.bmj.com

British National Formulary
https://bnf.nice.org.uk

European Medicines Agency
www.ema.europa.eu

Medline Plus
www.medlineplus.gov/

Northern California Comprehensive Thalassemia Center
www.thalassemia.com

Thalassaemia International Federation
https://thalassaemia.org.cy

UK Thalassaemia Society
https://ukts.org

UpToDate
www.wolterskluwer.com/en/solutions/uptodate

Fast Facts for Patients

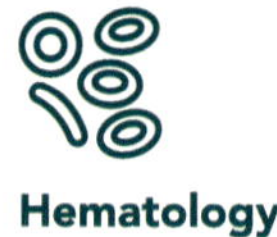

Hematology

Kevin HM Kuo MD MSc FRCPC
Associate Professor, Division of Hematology
University of Toronto, Canada

Medical writing support provided by Liz Woolf.

Made possible by a contribution from Agios. Agios did not have any influence on the content and all items were subject to independent and editorial review.

© 2023 in this edition, S. Karger Publishers Ltd.
ISBN: 978-3-318-07150-4

We'd like your feedback

How has this book helped you? Is there anything you didn't understand?
Do you still have any unanswered questions?
Please send your questions, or any other comments, to fastfacts@karger.com
and help readers of future editions. Thank you!

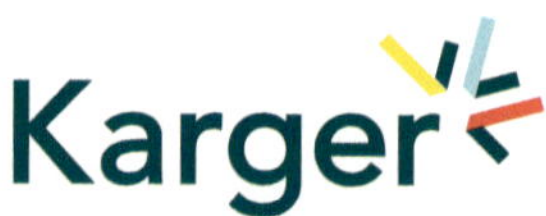

HEALTHCARE